SUPERFOOD JUICING

Over 75 Fresh and Healthy Recipes

Tina Haupert

CIDER MILL PRESS

BOOK PUBLISHERS

Kennebunkport, Maine

13-Digit ISBN: 978-1-60433-540-8
10-Digit ISBN: 1-60433-540-8

This book may be ordered by mail from the publisher. Please include $4.95 for postage and handling. Please support your local bookseller first!

Books published by Cider Mill Press Book Publishers are available at special discounts for bulk purchases in the United States by corporations, institutions, and other organizations. For more information, please contact the publisher.

Cider Mill Press Book Publishers
"Where good books are ready for press"
12 Spring Street
PO Box 454
Kennebunkport, Maine 04046

Visit us on the Web!
www.cidermillpress.com

Design by Emily Regis
Typography: Gill Sans, MrsEaves, and Avenir
All images used under license from Shutterstock.com.
Printed in China

1 2 3 4 5 6 7 8 9 0
First Edition

TABLE *of* CONTENTS

What Is Superfood Juicing   4

Getting Started   5

Choosing a Juicer   7

Simple Juices   11

Green Juices   27

Fruit Juice Blends   43

Vegetable Juice Blends   63

Energizing Juices   79

Index   95

WHAT IS SUPERFOOD JUICING?

Superfoods in the world of both natural and manufactured foods are the best of the bunch and rise above everything else on a nutritional level. They are the most nutritionally rich foods, as they contain the most vitamins, minerals, and phytonutrients per calorie. Superfoods include:

> **Dark leafy greens** like kale and collard greens
> **Brightly colored fruits and vegetables** like blueberries, beets, and pumpkin
> **Foods loaded with essential fatty acids** like raw nuts and chia seeds
> **Herbs and spices** like turmeric and ginger that contain powerful levels of antioxidants.

While the term *superfood* is not regulated, we do know that consuming lots of these nutrient-packed superfoods—while cutting back on commercially processed low-nutrient foods—helps support the natural metabolic processes of the body. Optimal health depends on the efficiency of our body's metabolic processes, including metabolism, digestion, absorption, and detoxification.

There's a significant difference between *Superfood Juicing* and commercial-processed juices. Home juicing these maximum-nutrient foods offers a supercharged dose of fresh and raw vitamins and minerals in your juice.

Juices and smoothies are easy and tasty ways to get more nutrient-packed superfoods in your diet. It's a fun way to be creative, experiment with different foods and flavors, and find what tastes good and makes you feel good, too.

— Breea Johnson, M.S., R.D., L.D.N.

GETTING STARTED

It's important to have the right tools
when it comes to making healthful smoothies and juice.
In this first chapter, you'll learn about what to look
for in a blender and a juicer, selecting the ingredients,
and best practices for producing the highest-quality
smoothies and juice.

It might seem like there's a lot to know, but the best
way to make delicious-tasting smoothies and juice
is to experiment with your favorite flavors and ingredients.
There's no right or wrong way to make them. As long
as you're including plenty of fruits, veggies, and other
nutrient-rich ingredients, your overall health
and wellness will benefit.

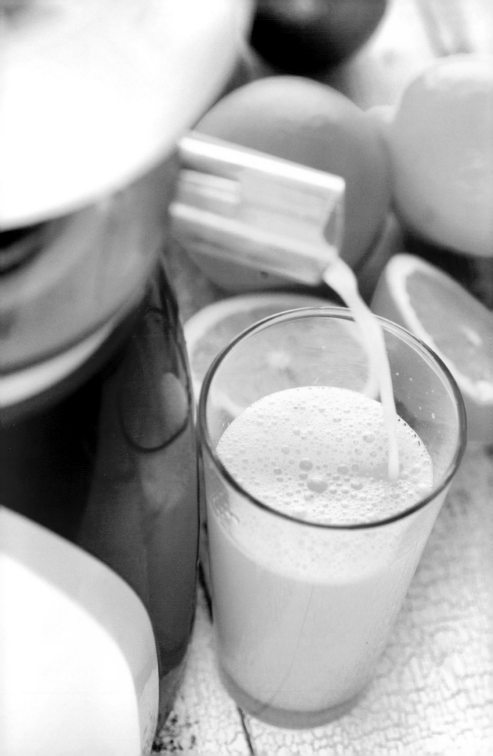

CHOOSING A JUICER

Electric juicers come in two main types: masticating (also known as cold press because they don't produce heat when they extract the juice) and centrifugal.

A **masticating juicer** works by smashing and crushing fruits and vegetables and then squeezing them through a fine, stainless steel strainer to produce juice. This type of juicer tends to be quieter and extracts more juice and nutrients because it generates less heat and friction. But masticating juicers also tend to be bulkier and more expensive than centrifugal juicers.

A **centrifugal juicer** has sharp, fast-spinning metal blades that shred the fruits and vegetables and then, using centrifugal force, separate the juice from the pulp, which are then separated into different containers. Some centrifugal juicers have an automatic pulp ejector that sends the pulp into a side container once the juice has been extracted, which makes cleanup easier and faster. Other centrifugal juicers have an extra-wide mouth that allows you to feed larger pieces of fruit and vegetables into the machine, which reduces the time spent cutting up produce to be juiced.

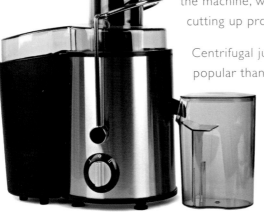

Centrifugal juicers tend to be more popular than masticating juicers because they're (sometimes) faster, easier to use and clean, as well as more affordable. But because the high-speed spinning blades inside the machines create heat, it can

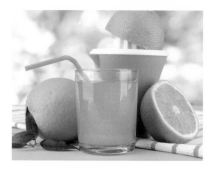

break down and destroy some of the enzymes in the fruits and vegetables that you are juicing. The heat also oxidizes the nutrients, which makes them less nutritious than a masticating (or cold press juicer) that produces no heat.

In the end, it's up to you which kind of juicer fits into your lifestyle and budget. If you're not too picky about getting the most nutrients or don't have a lot of money to spend, the centrifugal juicer might be for you. However, if you want to pack the most nutrients as possible into your body and don't mind spending a few extra bucks, go for the masticating (cold press) juicer.

No matter what you decide, consider the ease of use of the juicer you choose. If it's difficult to use or clean up, you won't use it often, which defeats the purpose of owning a juicer. Request an in-store demonstration, if possible, or watch videos reviews online to see the entire juicing process before purchasing.

Juicing Tips & Notes

- Use fresh, ripe, organic fruits, vegetables, and herbs for best results—that is, health benefits, nutrients, and taste.

- Wash and (if necessary) cut all fruits and vegetables before putting them into the juicer. If there are any bruised or damaged parts, remove them before juicing.

- Remove pits and seeds from fruit before juicing to prevent damaging machine parts.

- To help prevent pulp from clogging the machine, alternate soft/wet and hard/leafy produce whenever possible.

- Do not pour water, coconut water, or other juices directly into juicer unless specifically directed to do so.

- Make only as much juice as you will need and drink it right away because fresh juice will lose flavor and nutrients immediately after juicing.

- Be diligent about thoroughly cleaning your juicer after each use. This will not only help keep the machine in good working order but it can also help protect you from food poisoning caused by the growth of harmful bacteria left on the machine's parts.

- If the flavor of a juice is too intense, use water to lessen it. Water also increases the volume of the beverage, so it seems like you're drinking more. And, of course, water hydrates you!

- Because juicing machines and fresh produce vary so much and will give you different results, the juice recipes in this book produce one serving, which is equal to approximately 8 ounces of liquid.

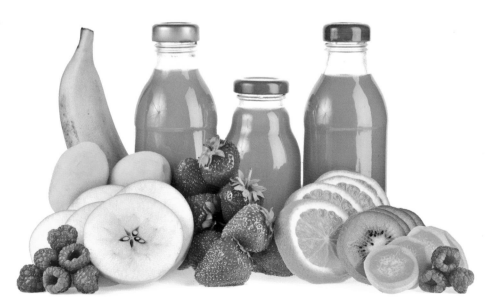

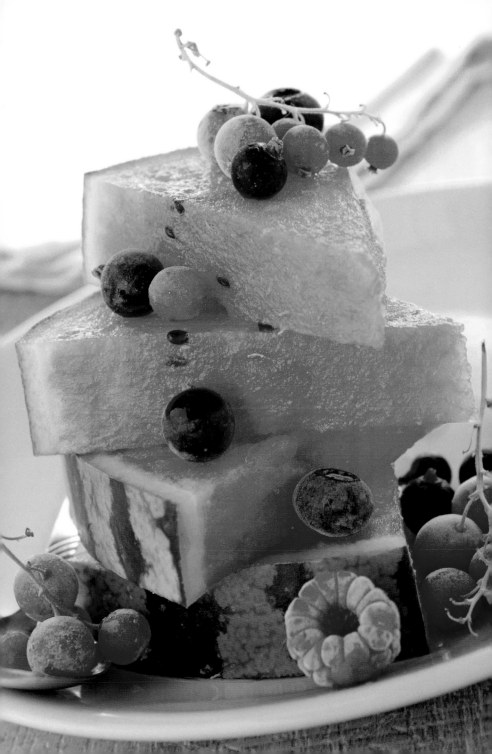

SIMPLE JUICES

The best part about making freshly pressed juice
is that it can be so simple. Even the juice of a single
vegetable or fruit is a tasty and healthy addition
to your diet.

Most of the recipes in this chapter have just three
ingredients, so you can juice them up in a matter
of minutes and still reap the health benefits of freshly
pressed juice from nutrient-rich produce.

You'll find traditional juice staples such as apple, orange,
pineapple, pear, lemon, grapefruit, and cranberry.
But this chapter also includes some ingredients you may
not have tried in juice before, such as cucumber, dandelion
greens, spinach, parsley, beets, carrots, cantaloupe,
and watermelon. Enjoy experimenting!

Oh, and if you're following a strict vegan diet,
all the juices in this book are vegan.

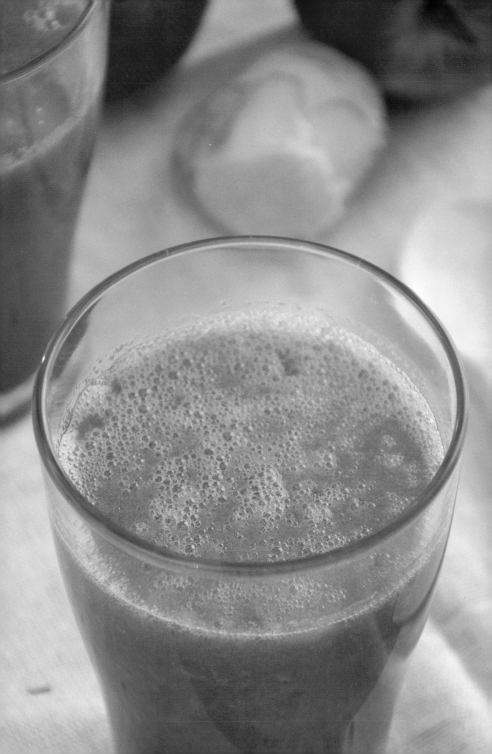

APPLE-BEET-PEAR (ABP) JUICE

Simple and delicious, this juice blend combines the flavors of earthy beets with sweet apple and pear and sour lemon to keep your taste buds guessing!

 I apple

 I pear

 2 beets

 Juice of ½ lemon

Combine all ingredients in a juicer. Pour juice into a glass or over ice and drink immediately.

Bonus Recipe

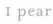 ## ZESTY APB JUICE
Add ¼-inch fresh ginger root while juicing.

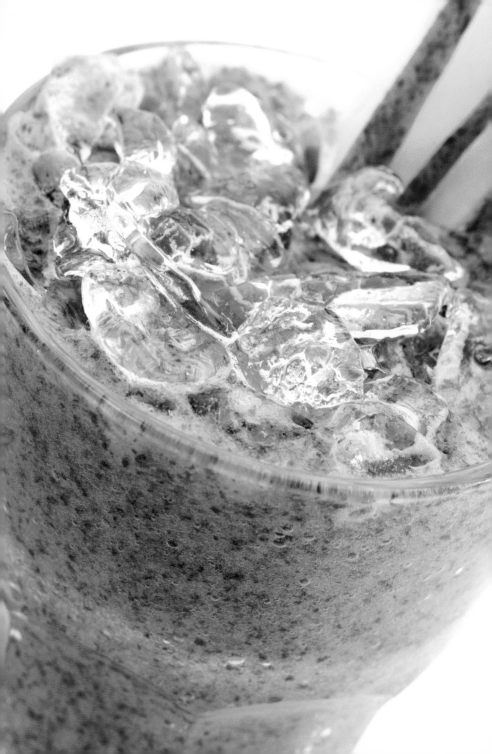

SPINACH-PEAR JUICE

Simple and nutritious, this juice comes together in matter of minutes, thanks to just three ingredients. Sweet pear combines with spinach and cucumber for a wonderful flavor and nutrient-rich combination that you'll want to drink again and again.

---

 3 pears

 2–4 ounces spinach

 ½ cucumber

Put ingredients into a juicer, alternating between spinach, chunked pears, and cucumber. Pour into a glass with ice, garnish with thin pear slices, and drink immediately.

Bonus Recipe

 ## PERFECT PEAR JUICE
Replace the ½ cucumber with a Granny Smith apple.

CARROT JUICE WITH A KICK

This isn't your regular glass of carrot juice! Thanks to apple, lemon, and ginger, this one has a little sweet, a little sour, and a whole lot of zip.

 6–8 carrots

 1 apple

 ½ lemon

 Fresh ginger root to taste

Combine all ingredients in a juicer. Pour juice into a glass or over ice and drink immediately.

Carrots provide your body with vitamin A as well as a host of other powerful health benefits, including healthy beautiful skin, cancer prevention, and anti-aging properties.

WATERMELON-BERRY BLEND

Here's a sweet berry blend for you! Pick your choice of fresh berries and then juice them with watermelon and red grapes. You're definitely in for a treat!

---

 2 cups raspberries or mixed berries

 1 cup chopped watermelon

 ½ cup red seedless grapes

Combine all ingredients in a juicer. Pour juice into a glass or over ice and drink immediately.

Bonus Recipe

 ## CANTALOUPE-BERRY BLEND
Replace watermelon with 1 cup of cantaloupe.

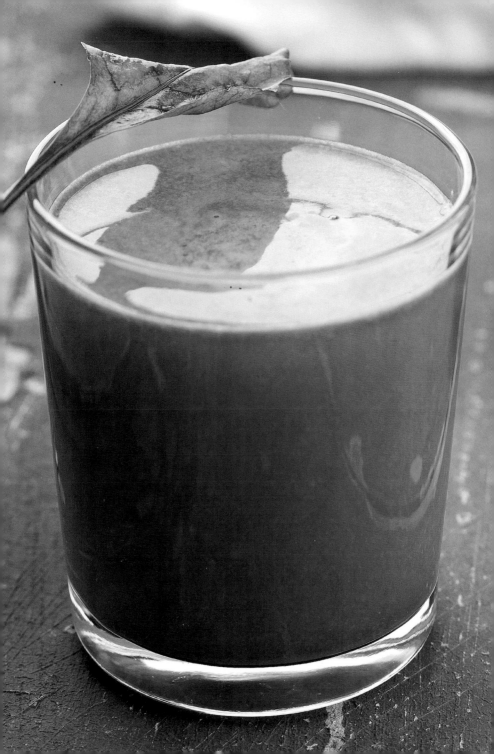

DANDY BLEND

Dandelion greens are a little bitter. But when combined with sweet apple and lemon citrus, they make a refreshing, mellow, and slightly sweet green juice.

---

 1 bunch dandelion greens

 2 apples

 ¼ lemon, peeled and segmented

Put ingredients into a juicer, alternating greens with chunked fruits and veggies. Pour into a glass or over ice and drink immediately.

Dandelion greens are loaded with calcium and iron—even more so than other greens. In addition, they have more protein per serving than spinach.

Bonus Recipe

 ## CARROT-DANDY BLEND
Replace the apples with carrots.

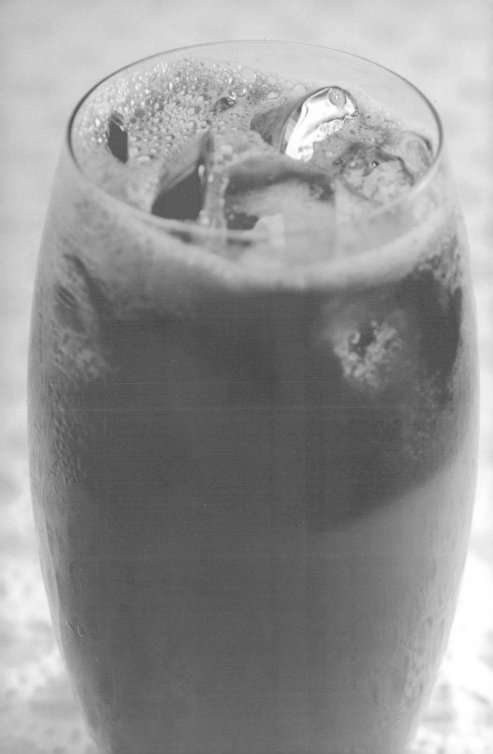

STRAWBERRY-ORANGE-PINEAPPLE JUICE

Pineapple, strawberry, and orange—all of my favorites in one juice!
This juice tastes a little tropical and a whole lot sweet!

 1½ cups of fresh pineapple, cut into chunks

 1½ cups strawberries

 1 orange or tangerine

Combine ingredients in a blender until smooth. Pour into a glass and enjoy immediately.

Bonus Recipe

 ## PINEAPPLE-APPLE-STRAWBERRY JUICE
Replace the orange with an apple.

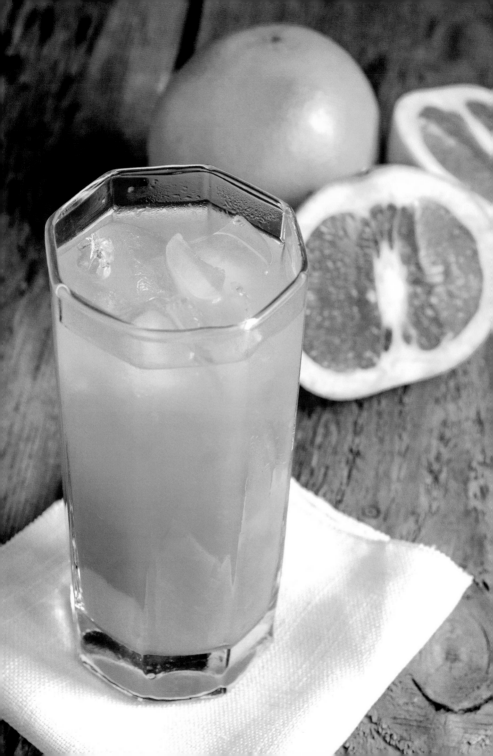

GRAPEFRUIT-CARROT-GINGER JUICE

Citrus and ginger are always an exciting flavor combination. This juice takes it one step further with sweet, earthy carrot.

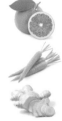

1 pink grapefruit, peeled and sectioned

6 carrots

Fresh ginger root to taste

Combine all ingredients in a juicer. Pour juice into a glass or over ice and drink immediately.

Bonus Recipe

GOLDEN DELICIOUS JUICE
Cut back on the number of carrots and add a Golden Delicious apple.

"A grapefruit is a lemon that had a chance and took advantage of it."

— OSCAR WILDE

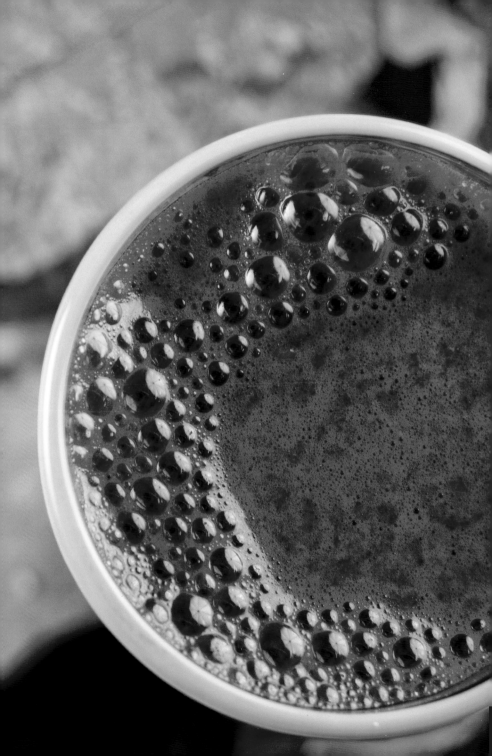

V3 JUICE

Made with just three different vegetables, this simple juice comes together in a matter of minutes and, boy, does it pack a nutritional punch. Packed with vitamin A, C, folate, fiber, and a whole slew of antioxidants, this juice will make you feel a tad bit healthier starting with the very first sip.

---

 2 beets

 5 carrots

 I cucumber

Combine all ingredients in a juicer. Pour juice into a glass or over ice and drink immediately.

Bonus Recipe

 ## APPLE-BEET JUICE
Use two carrots instead of five, and add an apple.

"Eat food. Not too much. Mostly plants."

— MICHAEL POLLAN

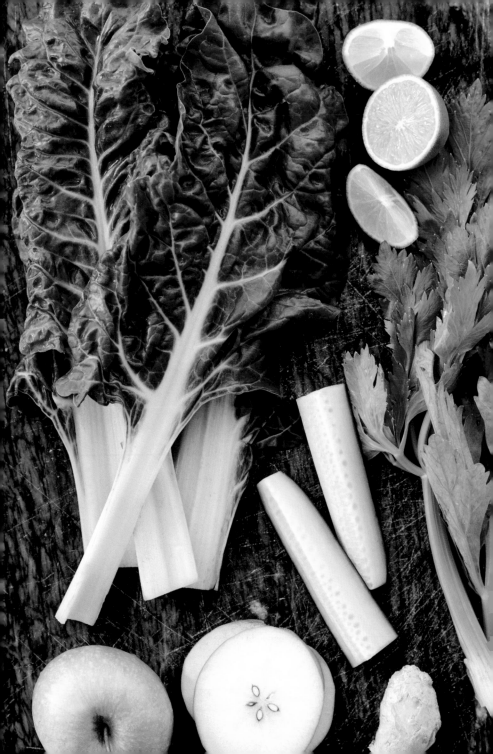

GREEN JUICES

Long before the term "superfood" was coined, Popeye was eating spinach for strength. Today we include it in our diets for a lot of reasons—everything from vitamin K for bone health, to vitamin C for cold-fighting powers, to lutein and zeaxanthin, which together act like sunscreen for the eyes.

The juices in this chapter have one obvious thing in common: They're green. They include spinach, kale, lettuce, or other greens—and don't hesitate to mix and match. Leafy greens—the darker the better—are a rich source of minerals, including iron, calcium, potassium, and magnesium, as well as vitamins K, C, E, and many of the B vitamins.

Mix in a little sweetness from fruit—like apples, melons, or citrus fruits. Add some spicy mustard greens, parsley, mint, or ginger. Or tone things down with some hydrating cucumber. Bottoms up!

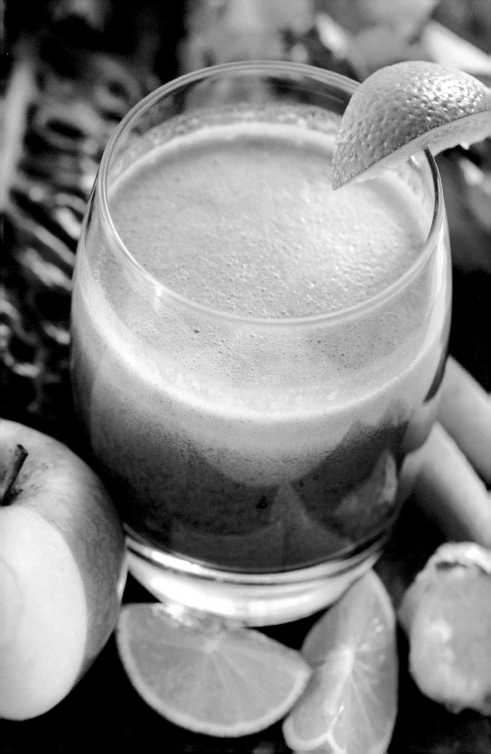

GREEN-AND-GO JUICE

This basic green juice will get you going!

---

 1 green apple

 4 ounces of fresh spinach

 4 celery stalks

 Lime wedge for garnish

Combine all ingredients in a juicer, alternating greens with chunked fruits and veggies. Pour juice into a glass or over ice and drink immediately.

Bonus Recipe

 ## ZESTY GREEN-AND-GO
For an extra kick, add fresh ginger root to taste.

Celery supplies essential vitamins A, C, and K, as well as the minerals folic acid and potassium, which helps regulate blood pressure.

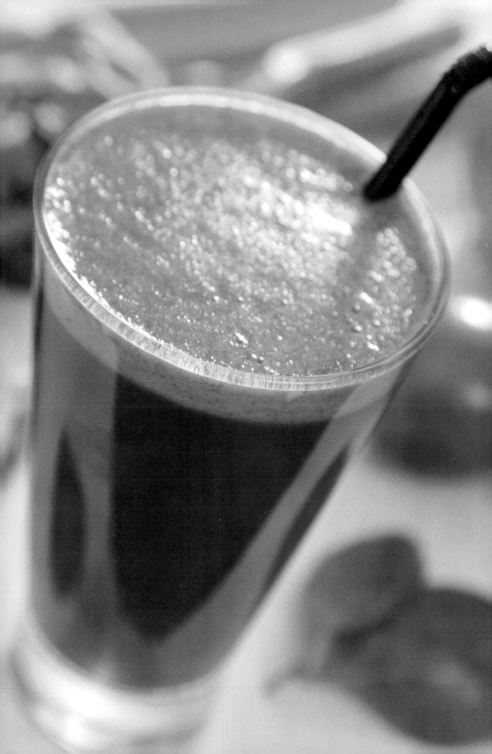

GREEN CITRUS JUICE

The ingredients in this mellow, green juice are straight-forward. But you'll be thoroughly impressed by their simple, refreshing flavors. This one is guaranteed to be a favorite.

 2 ounces baby spinach

 1 Granny Smith apple

 ¼ pink grapefruit

 6 celery stalks

Put ingredients into a juicer, alternating greens with chunked fruits and veggies. Pour into a glass or over ice and drink immediately.

Bonus Recipe

GREEN CITRUS KICK
For a little kick, add fresh ginger root to taste.

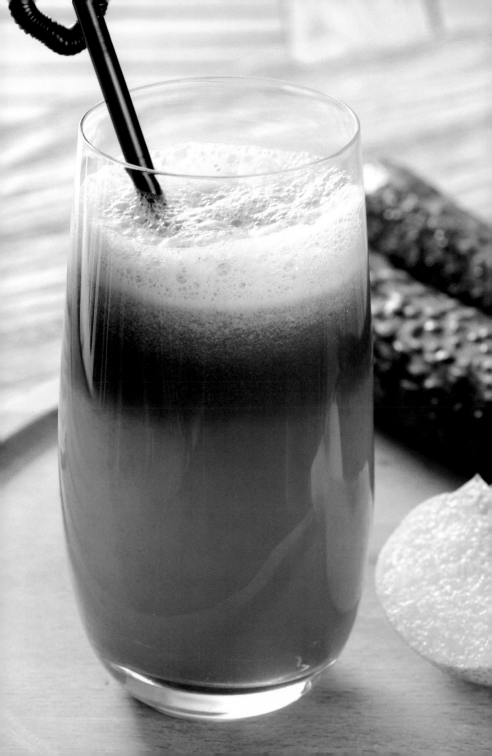

PEPPERY PEAR JUICE

There's nothing better than fresh arugula—that spicy, peppery taste is definitely something special. It combines with pear, cucumber, lemon, and ginger for a sweet, refreshing juice with a peppery zing.

---

 4 ounces fresh arugula

 1 pear

 1 cucumber

 ½ lemon, peeled and segmented

 Fresh ginger root to taste

Put ingredients into a juicer, alternating greens with chunked fruits and veggies. Pour into a glass or over ice and drink immediately.

Also known as "salad rocket," arugula is a rich source of folic acid and vitamins A and C. In addition, it's one of the best vegetable sources of vitamin K, which provides a boost for both bone and brain health.

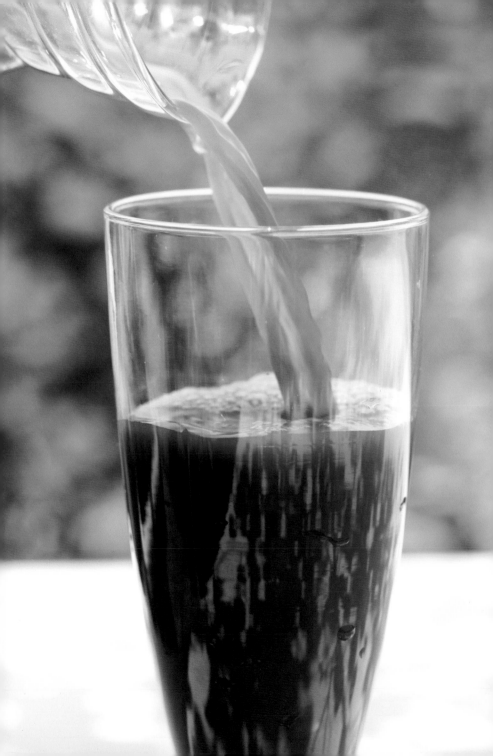

LEAFY GREEN GOODNESS JUICE

If you're craving some fresh greens in your diet, this juice is for you. You'll get a whole slew of antioxidants in this super green drink.

---

 2 ounces kale

 2 ounces spinach

 2 ounces of Swiss chard

 4 celery stalks

 1 cucumber

 ½ bunch parsley *optional*

Put ingredients into a juicer, alternating greens with chunked fruits and veggies. Pour into a glass or over ice and drink immediately.

Bonus Recipe

SWEET LOVE OF GREENS
For a sweeter version, swap out the celery stalks for a medium or large apple.

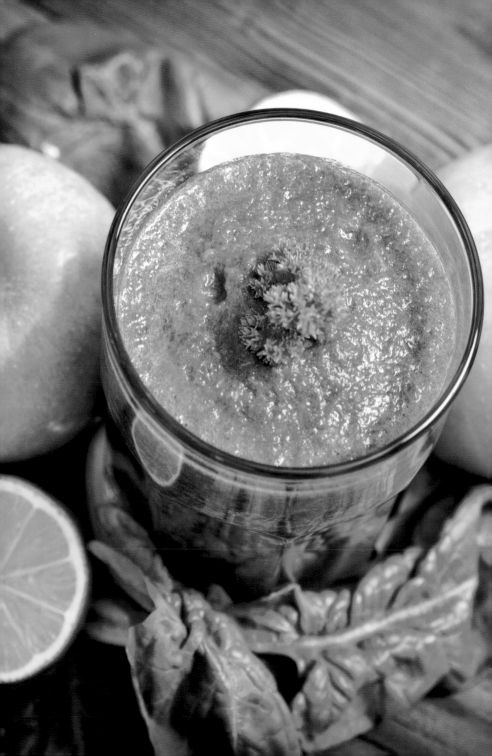

SWEET KALE JUICE

Superfood kale is loaded with vitamins K, A, and C, but it's also a tad bitter-tasting. Add some apple and watermelon, though, and you've got a sweet, smooth juice.

---

 4 ounces kale

 1 apple

 1 cup watermelon, cut into chunks

 Juice of ¼ lime

Put ingredients into a juicer, alternating greens with chunked fruits. Pour into a glass or over ice and drink immediately.

Bonus Recipe

 ## SWEET KALE TWIST
Use lemon juice instead of lime juice.

If greens such as kale or Swiss chard tend to be too bitter for you, try balancing the flavor with fresh lemon or lime. The acidity helps to neutralize the bitterness. Taste as you go: Try a good-size squeeze and then add more if needed.

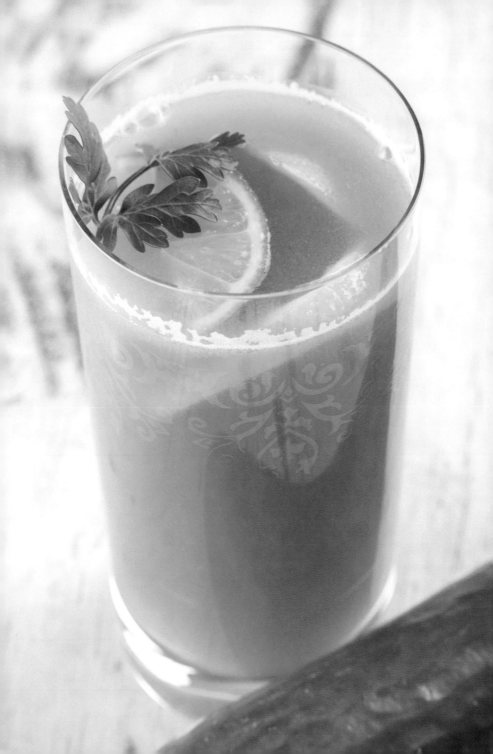

LIGHT 'N' GREEN JUICE

Sometimes you just feel like a light, refreshing, and hydrating green juice. Maybe dark leafy greens is a bit too bitter for your liking and you want something a little more mellow? If so, this juice is for you!

---

 4 ounces of romaine lettuce

 1 apple

 1 cucumber

 4 celery stalks

 ¼ lemon, peeled and segmented

Put ingredients into a juicer, alternating greens with chunked fruits and veggies. Pour into a glass or over ice, throw in a couple lemon or lime slices, and drink immediately.

Bonus Recipe

HOT & HYDRATING
Add a medium bunch of parsley before juicing. Finish with a few shakes of cayenne pepper and a teaspoon of hot sauce if you're feeling daring!

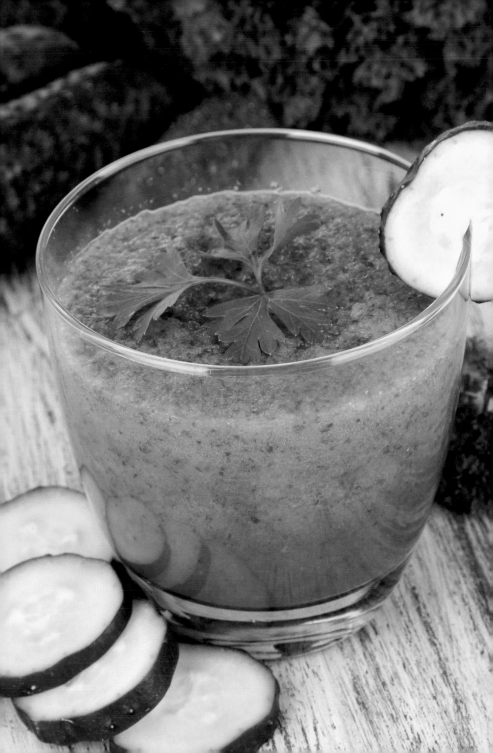

PARSLEY LOVERS' JUICE

Do you love the bold, peppery flavor of fresh parsley? If so, this juice is for you. Loaded with vital nutrients, this juice will wow you in more ways than one.

---

 4 ounces dark leafy greens of your choice

 I cucumber

 4 celery stalks

 ½ bunch to I bunch of flat leaf parsley

 ½ lemon, peeled and segmented *optional*

Put ingredients into a juicer, alternating greens with chunked fruits and veggies. Pour into a glass, garnish with a cucumber slice and a piece of parsley if you're feeling fancy, and drink immediately.

Parsley is rich in energy-producing chlorophyll and helps to build red blood cells, which increases energy levels.

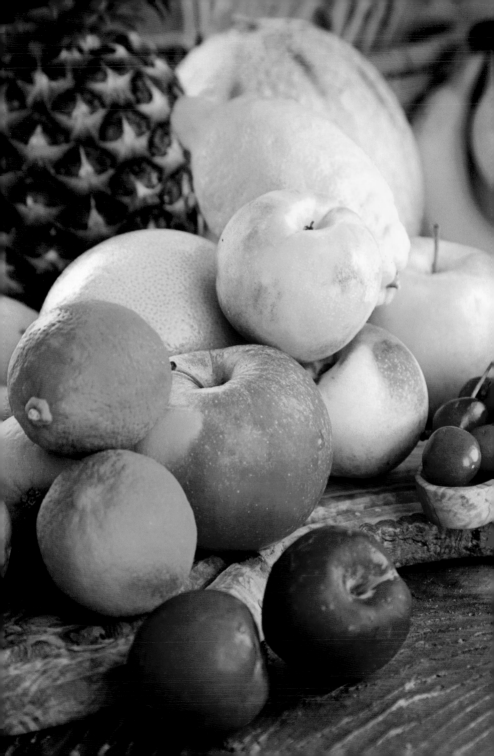

FRUIT JUICE BLENDS

Who doesn't love fresh-squeezed orange juice? Imagine how delicious a blend of fresh juices can be! These nutrient-dense juices are especially rich in vitamin C, which is essential for immunity. That's why an apple a day keeps the doctor away—because of its vitamin C content!

Juicing at home will give you the most nutrients, freshest juice for the price, as well as the flexibility to tweak the flavors to your liking. You won't have to worry about sugar, corn syrup, or artificial flavors sneaking in. But, for fruit fans not so keen on the veggies, you can easily sneak in some carrots or cucumber or even a green leaf or two.

The super-nutritious cast of characters here includes the whole berry family, citrus fruits, pineapple, mango, bananas, plums, and—for hydration—melons.

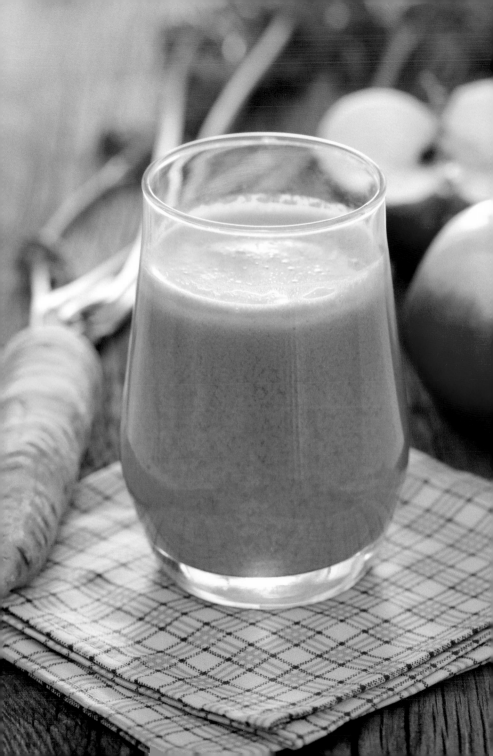

PINEAPPLE-GINGER-CARROT JUICE

This unique blend of tangy and sweet citrus juice packs a punch with a healthy dose of fresh ginger. You're guaranteed a refreshing taste experience.

 ½ apple

 I cup of fresh pineapple, cut into chunks

 4 carrots

 ¼-inch fresh ginger root

Combine all ingredients in a juicer. Pour juice into a glass or over ice and drink immediately.

Bonus Recipe

 ## PINEAPPLE-CARROT PUNCH
For a fruitier blend, use two carrots instead of four and add an apple.

Ginger is loaded with phytonutrients, which may help protect again a variety of diseases, including cancer and heart disease.

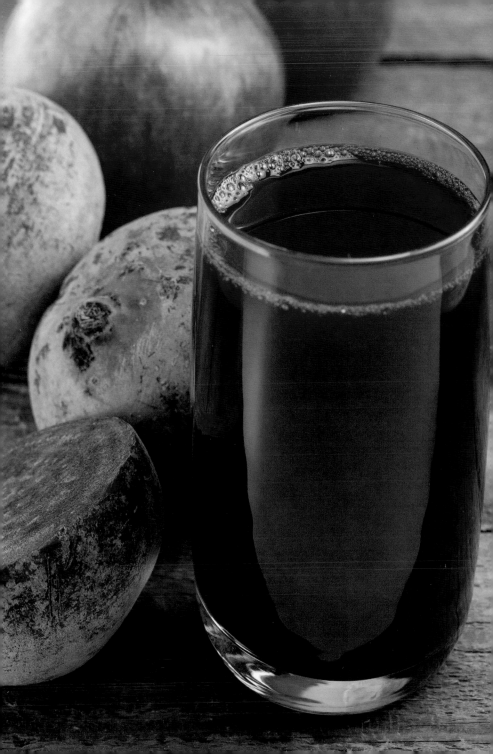

RED, RED JUICE

The ingredients in this juice combine to make a beautiful deep red. It's smooth and sweet, and likely a recipe that you will return to again and again.

---

 4 ounces spinach

 1 apple

 1 beet

 ½ cup blueberries

 ½ cucumber

Put ingredients into a juicer, alternating greens with chunked fruits and veggies. Pour into a glass or over ice and drink immediately.

Bonus Recipe

 ## BEET RED JUICE
Replace the spinach with two medium carrots.

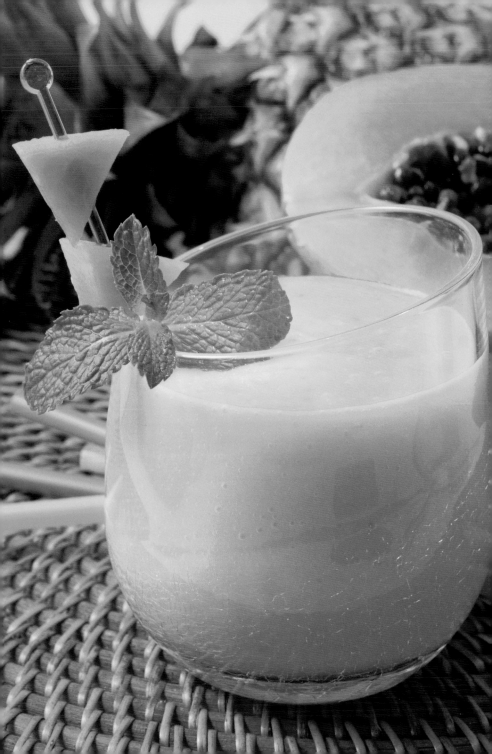

PINEAPPLE-PAPAYA PLEASER

A small papaya contains about 300 percent of the recommended daily amount of vitamin C. Pineapple, apple, and lemon also contain this immunity-boosting superstar, so you'll definitely get what you need for the day with this juice blend.

 I papaya, seeded and cut into chunks

 I cup pineapple, cut into chunks

 I apple

 ½ lemon, peeled and segmented *optional*

Combine all ingredients in a juicer. Pour juice into a glass or over ice and drink immediately.

Bonus Recipe

ISLAND OASIS
Drop the apple and lemon, use another cup of pineapple, and garnish with fresh mint and skewered fruit.

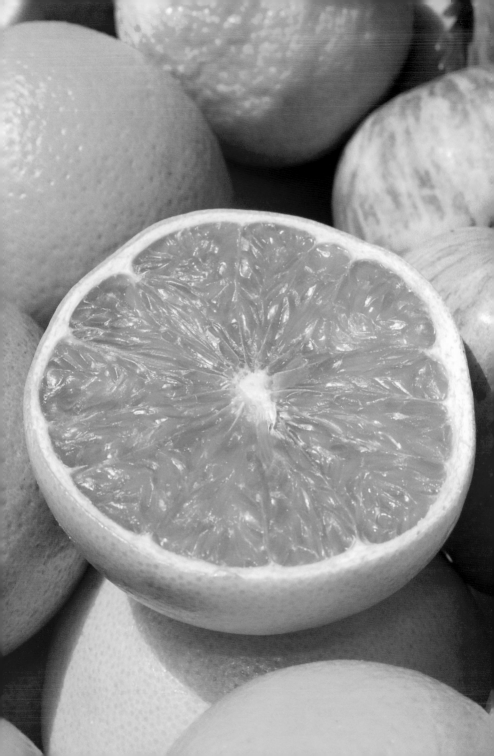

SOUR APPLE-GRAPEFRUIT JUICE

This isn't your typical glass of apple juice! This one is tangy and sour, thanks to the grapefruit.

---

 2 Granny Smith apples

 1 grapefruit, peeled

 ½ cup green grapes

Combine all ingredients in a juicer. Pour juice into a glass or over ice and drink immediately.

Bonus Recipe

KICK IN THE PANTS
Add fresh ginger root to taste. Tart with a zing!

The pectin in apples helps to lower both blood pressure and cholesterol.

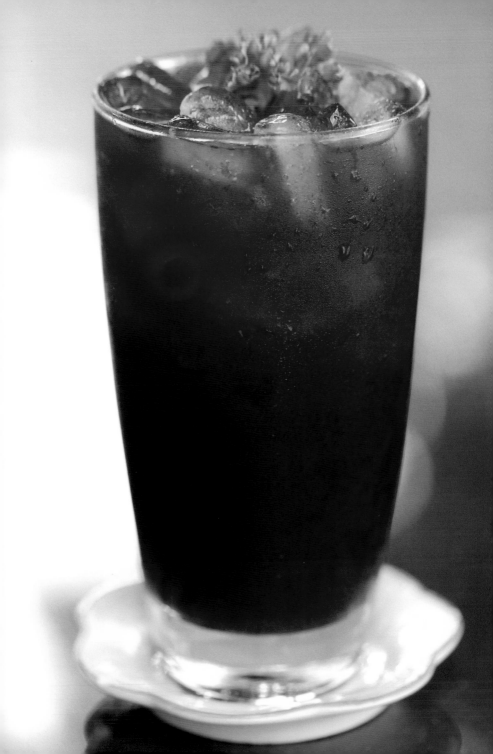

PLUM-BERRY JUICE

Plums and blueberries—what a delicious combination! When mixed with apple and cucumber, you'll enjoy an especially sweet and refreshing juice.

 3 plums, pitted

 1 cup blueberries

 1 apple

 ½ cucumber

Combine all ingredients in a juicer. Pour juice into a glass or over ice and drink immediately.

Bonus Recipe

 ## PLUM ASSIGNMENT
Replace the blueberries with blackberries, drop the cucumber, and add a squeeze of lime juice.

Plums are a good source of potassium, a mineral that helps manage high blood pressure and reduces the risk of stroke.

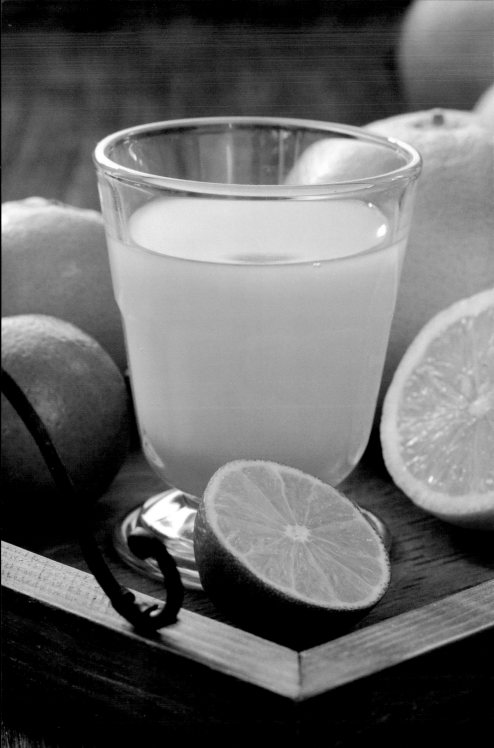

VITAMIN C BLEND

Vitamin C to the rescue! Feeling a little sluggish and need a natural boost? This juice is for you. Loaded with all sorts of vitamin-rich ingredients, this citrus blend tastes great and provides your daily dose of vitamin C.

---

 2 oranges

 2 kiwis, peeled

 ½ pink grapefruit, peeled and sectioned

 ¼ lime

 ¼ lemon, peeled and segmented

 Fresh ginger root to taste *optional*

Combine all ingredients in a juicer. Pour juice into a glass or over ice and drink immediately.

Bonus Recipe

 ## THE COLD FIGHTER
After juicing ingredients, add ½ tsp of cinnamon.

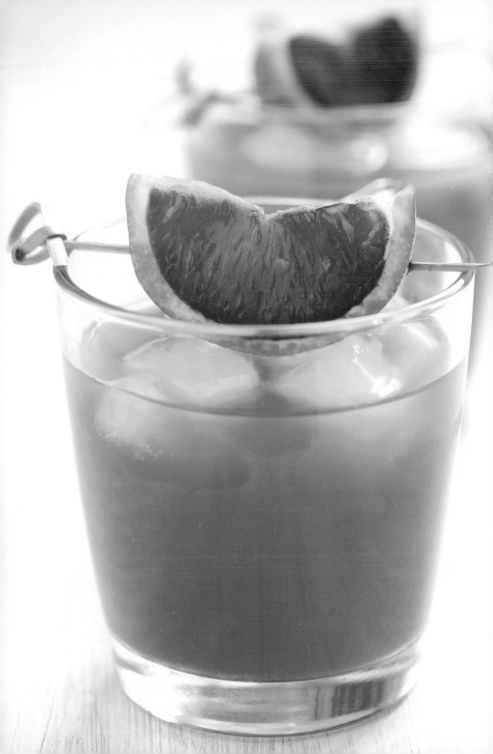

STRAWBERRY FIELDS

Fresh strawberry juice? You bet! This one is blended with cucumber, orange, and carrots for a delicious blend of fruits and veggies.

---

 2 cups strawberries, stems removed

 ½ cucumber

 1 blood orange, peeled and sectioned

 2 carrots

Combine all ingredients in a juicer. Pour juice into a glass or over ice, garnish with a skewered section of blood orange if you'd like, and drink immediately.

Who knew? Strawberries have more vitamin C than an orange!

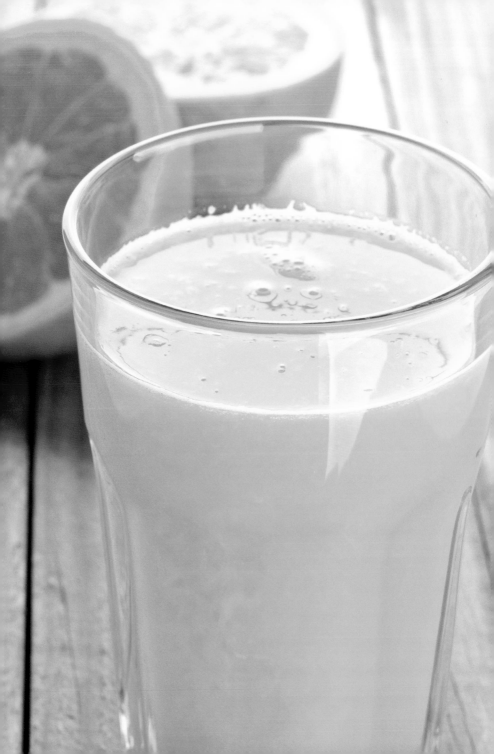

ORANGE CRUSH

This isn't your usual orange juice! Crisp apple, sweet cantaloupe, and fresh lemon combine for a flavor combination that will ignite your senses.

---

 2 oranges

 I apple

 I cup cantaloupe, cut into chunks

 ¼ lemon, peeled and segmented

Combine all ingredients in a juicer. Pour juice into a glass or over ice and drink immediately.

Bonus Recipe

ORANGE ZING
 For a juicy zing, add fresh ginger root before juicing.

CRAN-APPLE-ORANGE JUICE

Tart cranberries combine with sweet apple and orange for a tangy juice blend that you will love. Cranberries are a good source of vitamin C, E, and fiber as well as dental health.

---

 2 apples

 1 orange

 1 cup cranberries

Combine all ingredients in a juicer. Pour juice into a glass or over ice and drink immediately.

Bonus Recipe

CRAN-APPLE-STRAWBERRY JUICE
Instead of an orange, substitute 1 cup of fresh strawberries.

POMEGRANATE-BLUEBERRY CHILLER

On a hot summer day, sometimes all you want to do is chill out—with some nutrient-dense fruits, of course.

 ¾ cup blueberries

 ½ banana

 ¾ cup pomegranate juice

Combine fruit in juicer, then mix with pomegranate juice. Serve juice over ice cubes—or blend with ice. If you're making this chiller in the blender, feel free to use frozen blueberries and banana.

Bonus Recipe

 ## POMEGRANATE-STRAWBERRY CHILLER
Replace the blueberries with strawberries.

Pomegranate contains vitamins A, C and E, iron, and other antioxidants.

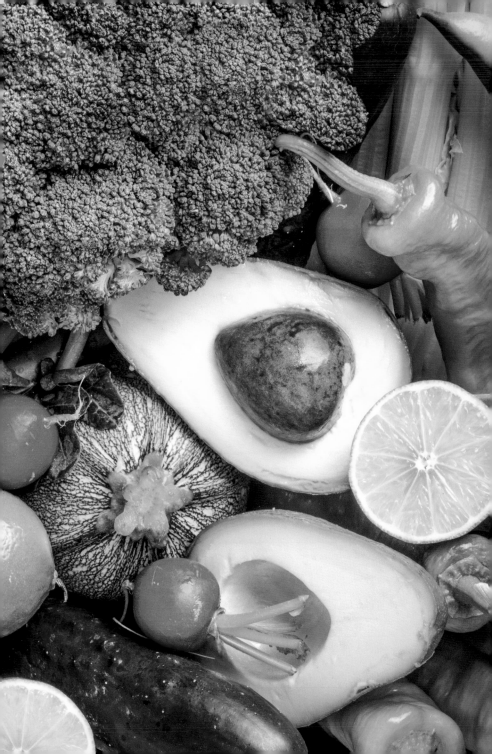

VEGETABLE JUICE BLENDS

If you're falling short on your daily intake of fresh vegetables, these juice blends are for you! Some of these juices have a half-dozen different veggie varieties in them. How's that for drinking the rainbow? Freshly pressed juice makes it easy to get a plethora of vitamins and minerals in your diet.

The majority of these vegetable juice blends tend to have an earthy, sometimes bitter flavor. You might love how these different vegetable tastes meld together, but if they're too strong for you, try diluting the juice with water or mellowing out the flavor by juicing an apple, pear, or cucumber along with the other ingredients. There's no wrong way to make juice. In fact, the only right way to make it is when you love the taste. Don't be afraid to experiment.

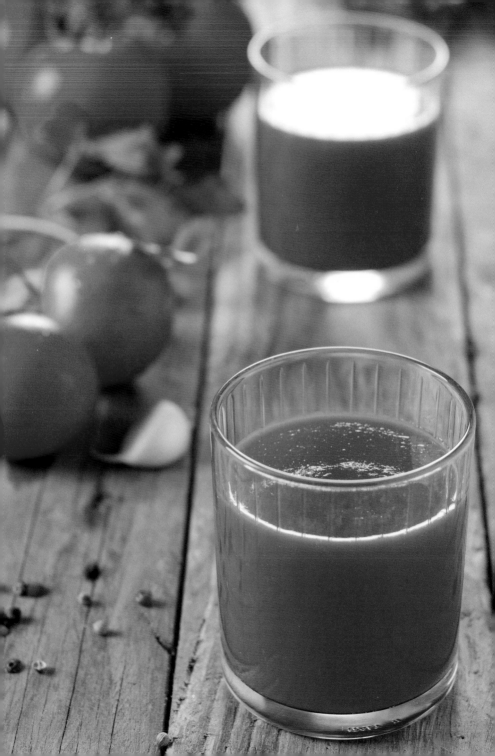

TOMATO-VEGGIE JUICE

Start your day on the right foot with this winning combination of vegetables. You'll get a whole slew of nutrients in each sip.

---

 3 medium tomatoes

 2 carrots

 2 celery stalks

 ½ lemon, peeled and segmented

 1 clove of garlic, peeled

 1 piece of horseradish to taste *optional*

 A pinch of sea salt

Combine all ingredients in a juicer. Pour juice into a glass or over ice and drink immediately.

Bonus Recipe

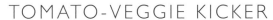

TOMATO-VEGGIE KICKER

 For an extra-spicy vegetable juice, add ½ jalapeño pepper before juicing.

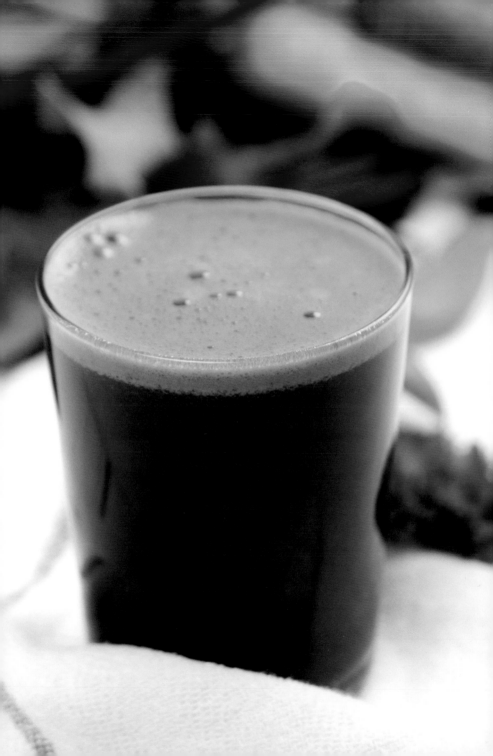

SPICY MUSTARD BLEND

If you like vegetable juice that bites back, you need to try this blend.

---

 4 ounces mustard greens

 1 medium tomato

 2 carrots

 4 celery stalks

 ½ lemon, peeled and segmented

 ½ jalapeño pepper (remove the seeds to make it less spicy)

Put ingredients into a juicer, alternating greens with chunked lemon and veggies. Pour into a glass and drink immediately.

Bonus Recipe

 ## HOUSE SALAD JUICE
For a less intense flavor, try fresh spinach, kale, or dandelion greens instead of mustard greens and leave out the pepper.

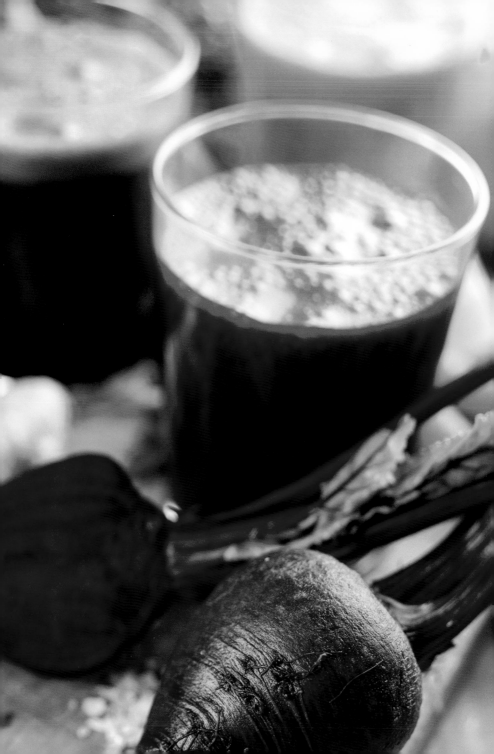

BEETLE JUICE

You'll love how you feel after drinking it this beet-based juice, loaded with essential vitamins and nutrients.

---

 4 ounces Swiss chard or spinach

 1 apple

 2 beets

 2 celery stalks

 ½ lemon, peeled and segmented *optional*

 Freshly ground pepper to taste *optional*

Put ingredients into a juicer, alternating greens with chunked fruits and veggies. Pour into a glass and drink immediately.

Bonus Recipe

GOLDEN BEETLE JUICE
For a color and flavor variation, use a golden beet instead of a red beet.

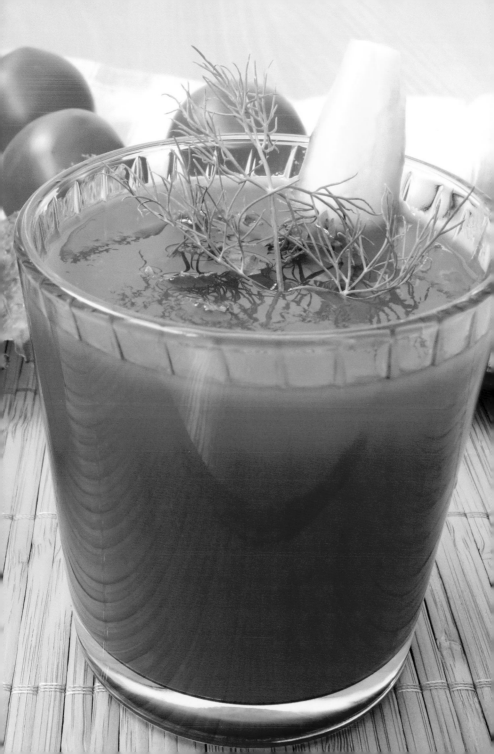

TOMATO-DILL JUICE

Fresh dill complements tomato so well in this juice. Add a touch of sea salt and freshly ground pepper for a savory juice full of flavor.

 4 tomatoes

 ½ cucumber

 1 bunch of dill

 Sea salt to taste

 Pepper to taste

Combine all ingredients in a juicer. Pour juice into a glass or over ice. Garnish with a lemon wedge, piece of dill, or celery sticks, and drink immediately.

Bonus Recipe

 ## MARY'S MOCKTAIL
Take some inspiration from the classic Bloody Mary cocktail and add three dashes of hot sauce.

Who knew? Chew fresh dill to help alleviate halitosis (bad breath)!

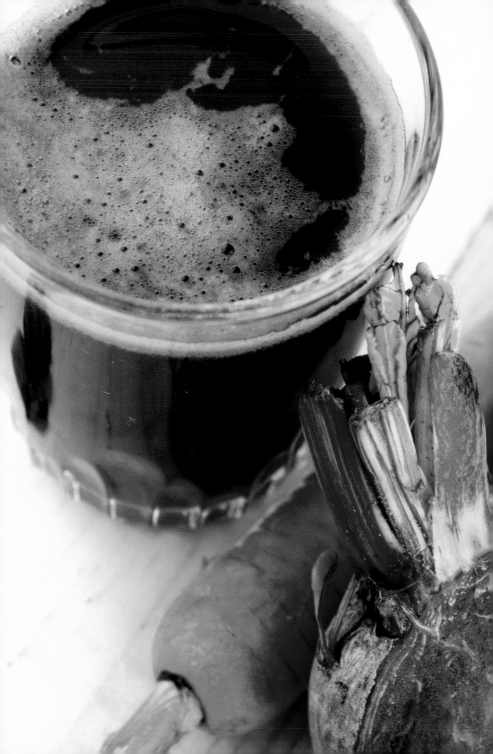

FEARSOME FOURSOME JUICE

These four vegetables pack some serious nutrients into one glass.
Combine them all together and you'll feel strong and fearless.

---

 2 beets

 4 carrots

 ½ medium sweet potato

 1 handful of dark leafy greens of your choice

Combine all ingredients in a juicer. Pour juice into a glass or over ice and drink immediately.

Beets contain a compound that helps fight inflammation and supports the body's natural detox processes. They're also a great source of folic acid as well as vitamin C, which is important for a strong immune system.

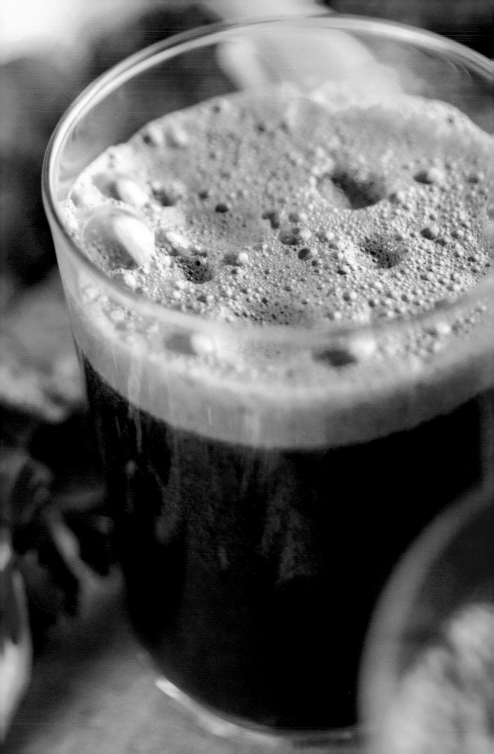

RAINBOW BRIGHT JUICE

Red, orange, yellow, and green—the colors in these ingredients will brighten up your day and start it off on the right foot.

---

 4 ounces kale (or spinach)

 2 cups pineapple, cut into chunks

 2 carrots

 1 beet

 ½ lemon, peeled and segmented *optional*

Put ingredients into a juicer, alternating greens with chunked fruits and veggies. Pour into a glass and drink immediately.

Bonus Recipe

 ## OVER THE RAINBOW
Add fresh mint leaves to taste.

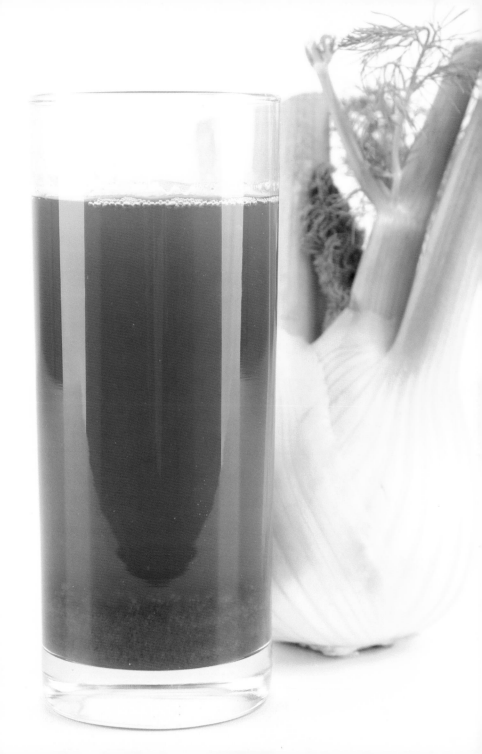

KALE-FENNEL-CARROT JUICE

Looking to try a new flavor in your juice? Try fresh fennel. It adds a fun, little zing to fresh juice. This juice includes nutrient-rich kale, carrots, and cucumber for a well-rounded and balanced juice.

 4 ounces kale

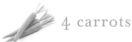 4 carrots

 1 cucumber

 ½ fennel bulb

Put ingredients into a juicer, alternating greens with chunked veggies. Pour into a glass and drink immediately.

Bonus Recipe

 ## KALE-FENNEL-APPLE JUICE
Replace the carrots with two apples and two stalks of celery.

Fennel was Thomas Jefferson's favorite vegetable.

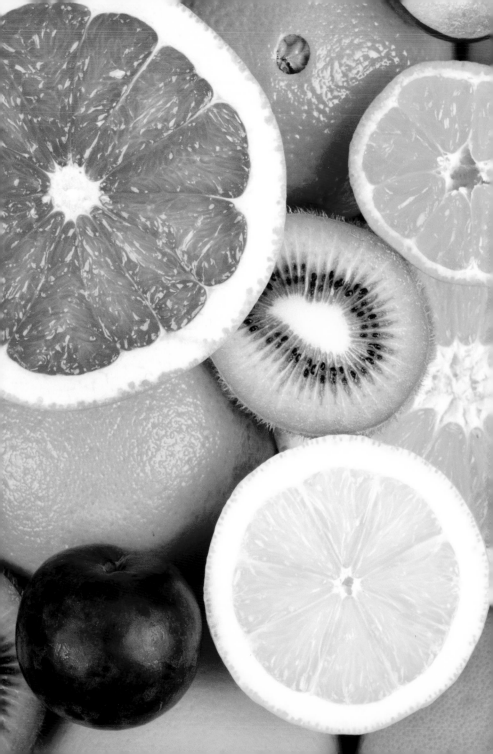

ENERGIZING JUICE

Are you dragging today? Lacking focus? Feel like taking a nap? Instead of reaching for a cup of coffee or brownie—both of which give you a temporary jolt of energy—try one of these energy-boosting juices. Drinking caffeine or eating a sweet treat may help you feel better quickly, but it's only temporary. The caffeine or sugar high usually wears off in an hour or so, which puts you right back where you started (and possibly feeling worse than before).

The recipes in this chapter are a natural remedy to help combat that sluggish feeling. They're filled with ingredients that will naturally boost your energy and get you going. Drink them first thing in the morning or in the afternoon to prevent that post-lunch slump.

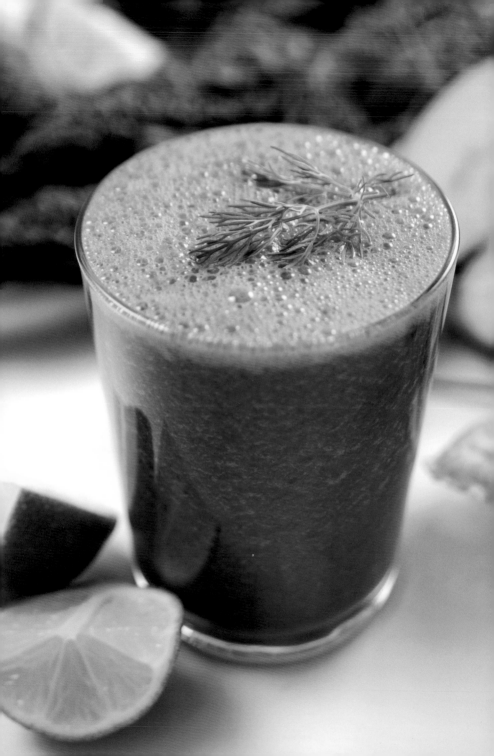

COCONUT-KALE-GINGER JUICE

Sweet coconut, bitter kale, and refreshing ginger might sound like a unique combination of ingredients, but they meld together so well in this juice. You'll get a natural pick-me-up starting with your very first taste!

 4 ounces kale

 2 Granny Smith apples

 ¼-inch fresh ginger root (or to taste)

 ½ cup coconut water

Put ingredients in a juicer, alternating greens with chunks of apples and slices of ginger root. Mix with the coconut water, pour into a glass, and drink immediately.

Bonus Recipe

 ## COCONUT-KALE-MINT JUICE
Not a fan of ginger? Skip it and add 8–10 leaves of fresh mint.

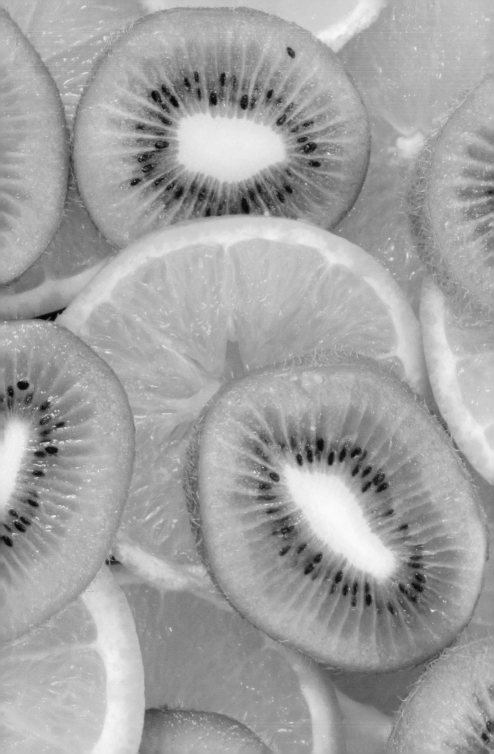

ORANGE-KIWI KICKER

This juice is loaded with nutrients, so you can start your day off on the right foot or drink it mid-afternoon for a natural energy boost.

 I orange, peeled and sectioned

 4 kiwis, peeled

 ¼ lemon, peeled and segmented

Combine all ingredients in a juicer. Pour juice into a glass or serve over ice.

Bonus Recipe

 ## ORANGE-KIWI BLAST
Add some fresh ginger root (¼ inch, or to taste).

Want a natural boost? Kiwis are rich in magnesium, a nutrient essential for converting food into energy.

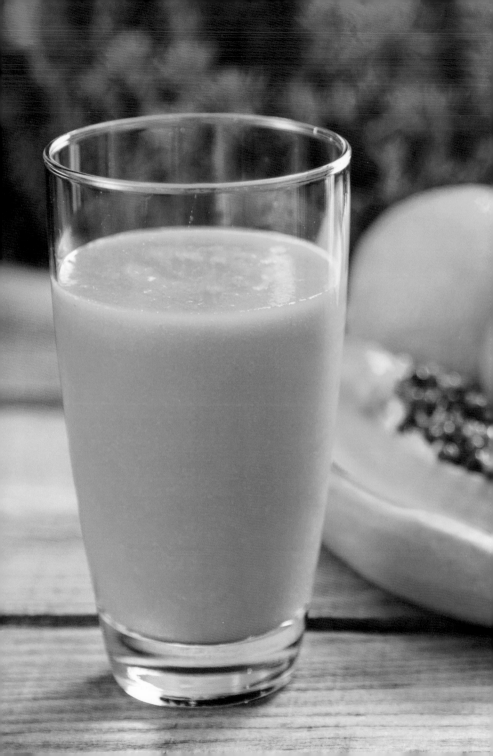

EVERYTHING ORANGE JUICE

There's so much healthy goodness in this super-orange juice!
Papayas are rich in vitamin C, potassium, and folate. They're also
full of vitamins A and E, which protect against heart disease.

---

 2 oranges, peeled and sectioned

 1 papaya, seeded and cut into chunks

 1 carrot

Combine all ingredients in a juicer. Pour juice into a glass
or serve over ice.

When buying papayas, look for ones that are mostly yellow
and give slightly to pressure. Avoid the green ones; they'll
never properly ripen.

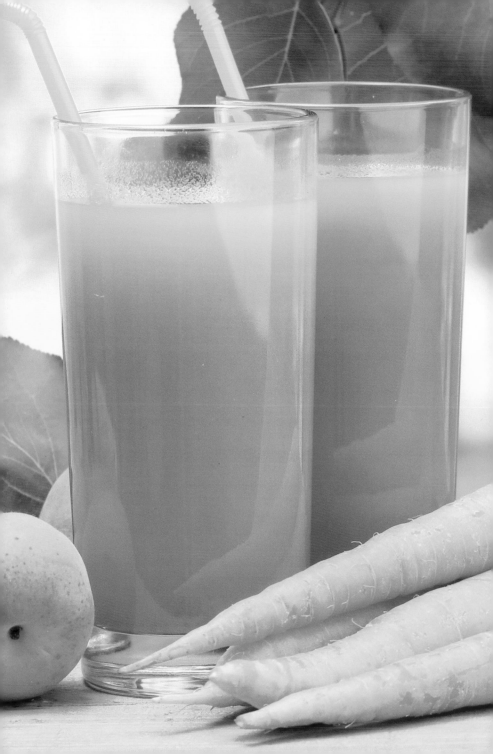

CARROT-APRICOT JUICE

You may not automatically think to pair apricots and carrots, but you'll be surprised by this delicious blend of flavors.

---

 4 fresh apricots

 6 carrots

 ½ cucumber

Combine all ingredients in a juicer. Pour juice into a glass or over ice and drink immediately.

Bonus Recipe

 ## CARROT TOP
For a spicy kick, add freshly grated ginger.

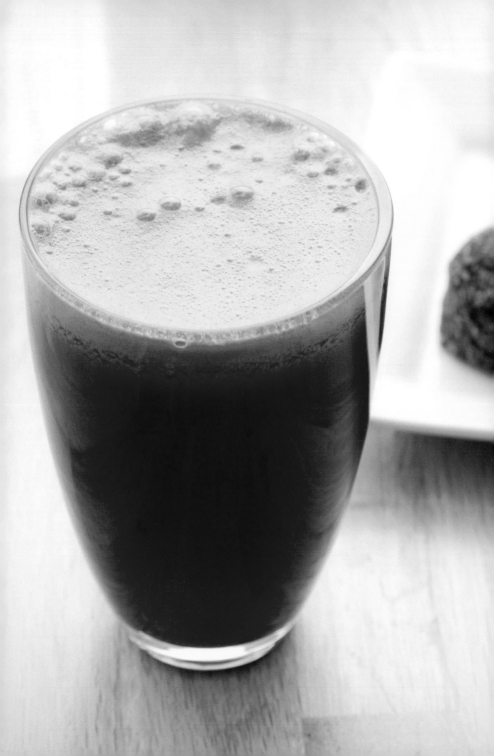

BEET-APPLE-GINGER JUICE

Rich in energy-boosting nutrients, this juice will make you feel full of life. Beets, apple, and ginger are an unforgettable combination that will liven your senses.

 3 apples

 3 beets

 Fresh ginger root to taste

Combine all ingredients in a juicer. Pour juice into a glass or over ice and drink immediately.

Bonus Recipe

 ## CARROT-APPLE-GINGER JUICE
Replace the beets with carrots.

WATERMELON-CUCUMBER COOLER

Perfect for hot summer days, this super-hydrating, cool, and refreshing juice is full of antioxidants and vitamins A and C. It's so delicious, it might just become your go-to juice of the summer!

 I cup watermelon, cut into chunks

 ½ cup honeydew melon, cut into chunks

 ½ cucumber

 ¼ lime

Combine all ingredients in a juicer. Pour juice into a glass or over ice and drink immediately.

Bonus Recipe

WATERMELON-CUCUMBER REFRESHER

For an extra-refreshing juice, add 8–10 mint leaves before juicing.

CHERRY-PINEAPPLE REFRESHER

Drinking a brightly-colored, nutrient-rich glass of juice is a great way to instantly give you a lift, and this juice does just that.

 1 Granny Smith apple

 2 cups pineapple, cut into chunks

 1 cup pitted cherries

Combine all ingredients in a juicer. Pour juice into a glass or over ice and drink immediately.

Bonus Recipe

CHERRY "TART"
Add ½ lemon, peeled and segmented, and 8–10 mint leaves.

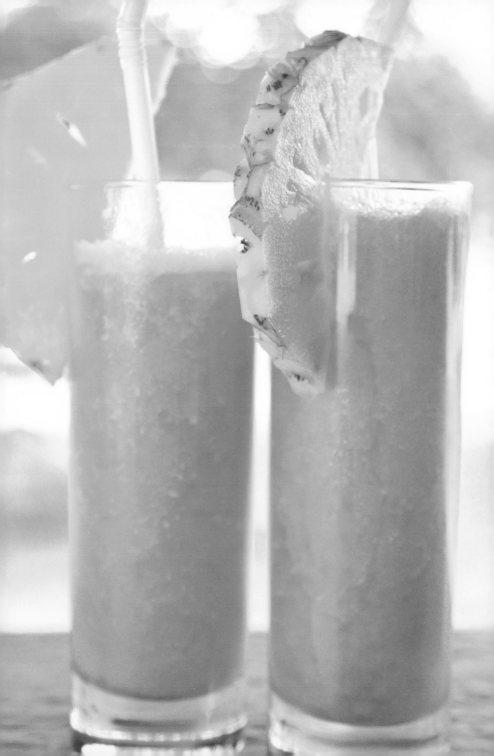

SUPER SUNBURST

When you're feeling lethargic and low on energy, skip the energy drink and reach for this sweet citrus blend. Instead of a quick boost that will leave you crashing sooner than later, this juice will give you long-lasting energy.

 2 oranges, peeled and sectioned

 1 cup pineapple

 1 sweet potato

Combine all ingredients in a juicer. Pour into a glass or over ice, garnish with a slice of pineapple and enjoy immediately.

Bonus Recipe

SUNBURST COLADA

 For a milky alternative, add ¼ to ½ cup of almond milk after juicing the other ingredients. Stir and enjoy.

COCONUT-LIME JUICE

Coconut water is incredibly hydrating, which will give you an instant boost if you're feeling a little parched. Juiced with fresh lime, apple, and spinach, it'll provide your body with a whole host of feel-good nutrients.

 1 lime

 ½ apple

 1 cup coconut water

 Handful of spinach *optional*

Put solid ingredients into a juicer, alternating greens with chunked fruits. Combine with the coconut water, pour into a glass, and drink immediately.

"It is health that is real wealth and not pieces of gold and silver."

— MAHATMA GANDHI

INDEX

Apple-Beet Juice 25
Apple-Beet-Pear Juice 13
Beet Red Juice 47
Beet-Apple-Ginger Juice 89
Beetle Juice 69
Berry Blend 17
Cantaloupe-Berry Blend 17
Carrot Top 87
Carrot with a Kick 16
Carrot-Apple-Ginger Juice 89
Carrot-Apricot Juice 87
Carrot-Dandy Blend 19
Cherry "Tart" 91
Cherry-Pineapple Refresher 91
Coconut-Kale-Ginger Juice 81
Coconut-Kale-Mint Juice 81
Coconut-Lime Juice 94
Cran-Apple-Orange Juice 60
Cran-Apple-Strawberry Juice 60
Dandy Blend 19
Everything Orange Juice 85
Fearsome Foursome Juice 73
Golden Beetle Juice 69
Golden Delicious Juice 23
Grapefruit-Carrot-Ginger Juice 23
Green Citrus Juice 31
Green Citrus Kick 31
Green-and-Go Juice 29
Hot & Hydrating 39
House Salad Juice 67
Island Oasis 49
Kale-Fennel-Apple Juice 77
Kale-Fennel-Carrot Juice 77
Kick in the Pants 51
Leafy Green Goodness Juice 35
Light 'N' Green Juice 39
Mary's Mocktail 71
Orange Crush 59
Orange Zing 59

Orange-Kiwi Blast 83
Orange-Kiwi Kicker 83
Over the Rainbow 75
Parsley Lovers' Juice 41
Peppery Pear Juice 33
Perfect Pear Juice 15
Pineapple-Apple-Strawberry Juice 21
Pineapple-Carrot Punch 45
Pineapple-Ginger-Carrot Juice 45
Pineapple-Papaya Pleaser 49
Plum Assignment 53
Plum-Berry Juice 53
Pomegranate-Blueberry Chiller 61
Pomegranate-Strawberry Chiller 61
Rainbow Bright Juice 75
Red, Red Juice 47
Sour Apple-Grapefruit Juice 51
Spicy Mustard Blend 67
Spinach-Pear Juice 15
Strawberry Fields 57
Strawberry-Orange-Pineapple Juice 21
Sunburst Colada 93
Super Sunburst 93
Sweet Kale Juice 37
Sweet Kale Twist 37
Sweet Love of Greens 35
The Cold Fighter 55
Tomato-Dill Juice 71
Tomato-Veggie Juice 65
Tomato-Veggie Kicker 65
V3 Juice 25
Vitamin C Blend 55
Watermelon-Berry Blend 17
Watermelon-Cucumber Cooler 90
Watermelon-Cucumber Refresher 90
Zesty ABP Juice 13
Zesty Green-and-Go 29

ABOUT CIDER MILL PRESS
BOOK PUBLISHERS

Good ideas ripen with time. From seed to harvest, Cider Mill Press brings fine reading, information, and entertainment together between the covers of its creatively crafted books. Our Cider Mill bears fruit twice a year, publishing a new crop of titles each spring and fall.

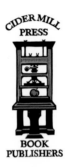

Visit us on the Web at
www.cidermillpress.com
or write to us at
12 Spring Street
PO Box 454
Kennebunkport, Maine 04046